MIND DIET VEGAN COOKBOOK FOR BEGINNERS

Mindful Vegan Cuisine: 61 Nourishing Recipes for Cognitive Health

By

DR.Ashley McGrane

Table of contents

<u>**Chapter 1: Introduction to Mind Diet Vegan Lifestyle**</u>

<u>**Overview of the Mind Diet and its benefits**</u>

The Mind Diet, short for the Mediterranean-DASH Diet Intervention for Neurodegenerative Delay, is a nutritional approach designed to promote brain health and reduce the risk of cognitive decline. It combines aspects of the Mediterranean and DASH (Dietary Approaches to Stop Hypertension) diets, both of which have been linked to numerous health benefits. The Mind Diet emphasizes the consumption of nutrient-dense foods, including fruits, vegetables, whole grains, nuts, and fish, while limiting the intake of red meat, sweets, and processed foods. These dietary choices are rich in antioxidants, omega-3 fatty acids, and other nutrients that have been associated with improved cognitive function and a lower risk of neurodegenerative diseases, such as Alzheimer's. The diet also encourages moderate alcohol intake, particularly red wine, and emphasizes the importance of staying physically active. Regular adherence to the Mind Diet has shown promising results in various studies, suggesting that it may contribute to better cognitive aging, memory retention, and overall brain health. The focus on a balanced and diverse array of nutrient-rich foods makes the Mind Diet not only beneficial for cognitive function but also for overall cardiovascular health, providing a holistic approach to well-being.

The Mind Diet places a strong emphasis on specific food groups known for their cognitive benefits. Fruits and vegetables, particularly berries and leafy greens, are rich in antioxidants that help combat oxidative stress and inflammation, key contributors to neurodegenerative diseases. Additionally, the inclusion of whole grains provides a steady supply of energy and essential nutrients for optimal brain function.

Nuts and seeds, another integral part of the Mind Diet, offer a source of healthy fats, including omega-3 fatty acids, which are crucial for brain health. Fatty fish, such as salmon and trout, are also recommended due to their omega-3 content, known for supporting cognitive function and protecting against age-related cognitive decline.

The diet promotes lean protein sources, like poultry and legumes, while limiting red meat and processed meats. Reducing the intake of saturated and trans fats supports heart health, indirectly benefiting cognitive function by improving blood flow to the brain.

Moderate alcohol consumption, particularly red wine, is a distinctive feature of the Mind Diet. Some studies suggest that the antioxidants in red wine, such as resveratrol, may have neuroprotective properties. However, it's crucial to note that excessive alcohol intake can have detrimental effects, so moderation is key.

In addition to dietary recommendations, the Mind Diet encourages regular physical activity. Exercise has been linked to improved cognitive function and a reduced risk of cognitive decline. The combination of a nutrient-rich diet and an active lifestyle creates a comprehensive approach to promoting brain health and overall well-being.

It's important to consult with healthcare professionals before making significant changes to your diet, especially if you have existing health conditions. The Mind Diet, with its focus on a balanced and varied array of foods, offers a sustainable and enjoyable approach to supporting cognitive health.

The MIND diet, developed by researchers at Rush University Medical Center, specifically targets brain health by incorporating foods associated with cognitive function and longevity. Here are some key aspects:

1. <u>Emphasis on Brain-Boosting Foods:</u>

   - <u>Leafy Greens:</u> Regular consumption of leafy greens like kale and spinach is encouraged, as they are rich in vitamins and minerals linked to brain health.

- <u>Berries:</u> Blueberries, in particular, are considered beneficial due to their high levels of antioxidants, which may help protect the brain from oxidative stress.

2. <u>Inclusion of Healthy Fats:</u>

   - <u>Olive Oil:</u> The diet promotes the use of olive oil as a primary source of healthy fats, known for its anti-inflammatory properties.

   - <u>Nuts and Fish:</u> Incorporating nuts, especially walnuts, and fatty fish like salmon provides omega-3 fatty acids, essential for brain function.

3. <u>Whole Grains and Legumes:</u>

   -<u>Whole Grains:</u> Foods such as brown rice and quinoa are included for their complex carbohydrates, providing sustained energy and supporting overall health.

   - <u>Legumes:</u> Beans and lentils are encouraged for their fiber content and contribution to heart health.

4. <u>Moderate Red Wine Consumption:</u>

   - Moderate consumption of red wine is suggested due to its potential cardiovascular benefits and the presence of certain compounds that may support brain health.

5. Limitation of Certain Foods:

   - Reduced Intake of Red Meat: The diet recommends limiting red meat consumption, as high intake has been associated with increased risk of neurodegenerative diseases.

   - Restriction of Processed Foods: Highly processed and sugary foods are discouraged.

6. Meal Structure:

   - Regular, Balanced Meals: The MIND diet promotes a well-balanced approach to meals, focusing on a variety of nutrient-dense foods.

Research has shown that adherence to the MIND diet may contribute to a lower risk of cognitive decline and neurodegenerative diseases. However, it's important to note that individual responses to diet can vary, and the MIND diet should be part of an overall healthy lifestyle.

Explanation of the vegan approach and its impact on cognitive health

The vegan approach, characterized by the exclusion of all animal-derived products from one's diet, has gained popularity not only for ethical and environmental reasons but also for its potential impact on health, including cognitive well-being.

A well-planned vegan diet can provide a rich array of nutrients that are beneficial for brain health. Fruits, vegetables, whole grains, nuts, seeds, and legumes, staples of a vegan diet, are packed with antioxidants, vitamins, and minerals that contribute to the reduction of oxidative stress and inflammation, which are associated with cognitive decline. Omega-3 fatty acids, crucial for brain function, can be obtained from plant-based sources such as flaxseeds, chia seeds, and walnuts. The absence of saturated fats in many plant-based foods aligns with cardiovascular health, indirectly benefiting cognitive function by promoting proper blood flow to the brain. While a vegan diet has the potential to support cognitive health, careful planning is essential to ensure adequate intake of nutrients like vitamin B12, iron, zinc, and calcium, which are often found in animal products. Supplementation may be necessary for certain nutrients.

In addition to the nutritional aspects, the vegan lifestyle can offer other potential cognitive health benefits. Some studies suggest that plant-based diets may be associated with a lower risk of certain chronic conditions, such as heart disease and type 2 diabetes, which are linked to cognitive decline. By reducing the risk of these conditions, a vegan diet may indirectly contribute to maintaining cognitive function over the long term.

Moreover, the vegan approach often encourages the consumption of whole, unprocessed foods, promoting a diet rich in fiber and phytonutrients. This can positively impact gut health, as the microbiome plays a crucial role in various aspects of health, including cognitive function. The gut-brain axis, a bidirectional communication system between the gut and the brain, is increasingly recognized for its influence on mood, cognition, and overall mental well-being. A plant-based diet that supports a diverse and healthy gut microbiome may contribute to these positive effects.

On the flip side, it's essential to be mindful of potential nutrient deficiencies that can arise with a vegan diet. Vitamin B12, for instance, is primarily found in animal products, and its deficiency can lead to neurological issues. Vegans may need to supplement or consume fortified foods to ensure an adequate intake of B12. Additionally, iron and zinc absorption from plant-based sources can be less efficient than from animal sources, necessitating careful food choices and, in some cases, supplementation.

Ultimately, while a well-planned vegan diet can offer numerous health benefits, including potential cognitive advantages.

Chapter 2: Essentials of Mindful Eating

Guidance on mindful eating practices

Mindful eating practices can enhance the benefits of the Mind Diet for vegans by promoting a deeper connection between food and overall well-being. Here are some guidance tips for incorporating mindful eating into a Mind Diet with a vegan approach:

1. <u>Savor Each Bite:</u> Take the time to appreciate the flavors, textures, and aromas of your food. Eating slowly allows you to savor each bite and fosters a greater sense of satisfaction, reducing the likelihood of overeating.

2. <u>Mindful Meal Preparation:</u> Engage in the process of preparing your meals. Connect with the ingredients, appreciate their colors and textures. This not only enhances your cooking experience but also reinforces a mindful connection to the food you're about to consume.

3. <u>Listen to Hunger and Fullness Cues:</u> Pay attention to your body's hunger and fullness signals. Before eating, assess your level of hunger, and while eating, pause periodically to check if you're comfortably satisfied. This helps in preventing overeating and promotes a healthier relationship with food.

4. <u>Limit Distractions:</u> Minimize distractions during meals. Turn off screens, put away electronic devices, and create a calm environment. This allows you to focus on the sensory experience of eating and fosters a mindful awareness of the nourishment you're providing your body.

5. <u>Gratitude for Plant-Based Choices:</u> Cultivate gratitude for the abundance of plant-based foods that contribute to your well-being. Reflect on the positive impact of your food choices on both your health and the environment, reinforcing a sense of purpose and satisfaction in your dietary decisions.

6. <u>Variety and Balance:</u> Embrace the variety of plant-based foods available to you. Aim for a colorful plate with a diverse range of fruits, vegetables, whole grains, legumes, nuts, and seeds. This not only ensures a well-rounded nutrient intake but also adds vibrancy to your meals.

7. <u>Mindful Snacking:</u> If you engage in snacking, do so mindfully. Choose nutrient-dense snacks like fresh fruits, raw veggies, or a handful of nuts. Be conscious of portion sizes and enjoy each bite consciously.

8. <u>Cultivate Awareness of Emotional Eating:</u> Be mindful of emotional triggers that may lead to overeating. Instead of using food as a coping mechanism, explore alternative ways to address emotional needs, such as practicing relaxation techniques or engaging in activities you enjoy.

9. <u>Mindful Hydration:</u> In addition to mindful eating, pay attention to your hydration. Opt for water, herbal teas, or infused water with slices of fruits and herbs. Being mindful of your liquid intake contributes to overall well-being and can complement the positive effects of a plant-based diet.

10. <u>Environmental Awareness:</u> Consider the environmental impact of your food choices. Mindful eating extends beyond personal well-being to include the broader ecosystem. Choose sustainably sourced, locally produced, and minimally packaged vegan foods when possible, aligning your choices with ethical and ecological considerations.

11. <u>Grains and Legumes Mindfulness:</u> Acknowledge the importance of grains and legumes in a vegan Mind Diet. These staples provide essential nutrients and are versatile in cooking. Experiment with various whole grains and legumes mindfully, appreciating the diverse textures and flavors they bring to your meals.

12. <u>Mindful Cooking Techniques:</u> Explore different cooking methods mindfully. Whether you're sautéing, roasting, or steaming, be present in the process. This enhances your connection to the food you're preparing and allows you to make conscious choices about the flavors and nutritional content of your meals.

13. <u>Intuitive Eating:</u> Practice intuitive eating by listening to your body's signals and responding appropriately. Pay attention to hunger and fullness cues, and let your body guide your eating patterns. This approach fosters a healthier relationship with food and promotes a sustainable, balanced dietary lifestyle.

14. <u>Mindful Social Eating:</u> When dining with others, be present in the social aspect of sharing a meal. Engage in conversation, savor the companionship, and appreciate the communal experience of enjoying plant-based dishes together. This enhances the overall satisfaction derived from the meal.

15. <u>Reflect on Food Origins:</u> Take a moment to reflect on the origins of your food. Consider the journey of plant-based ingredients from the farm to your plate. This awareness can deepen your connection to the food you consume and foster a sense of appreciation for the efforts involved in sustainable and ethical food production.

16. <u>Mindful Dessert Choices:</u> If you enjoy vegan desserts, approach them with mindfulness. Choose desserts made from whole, minimally processed ingredients, and savor them in moderation. This allows you to satisfy your sweet cravings while maintaining a health-conscious approach to indulgence.

By incorporating these mindful eating practices into the Mind Diet with a vegan focus, individuals can not only optimize their nutritional intake but also cultivate a more mindful and sustainable approach to their dietary habits, promoting both physical and mental well-being.

Importance of savoring flavors and textures.

Savoring flavors and textures holds paramount importance for Mind Diet vegans, as it not only enhances the overall dining experience but also contributes to the nutritional and psychological aspects of their plant-based lifestyle. By consciously appreciating the diverse flavors and textures present in a vegan diet, individuals can derive increased satisfaction from meals, making the transition to this dietary approach more enjoyable and sustainable.

The Mind Diet for vegans places a strong emphasis on a wide variety of plant-based foods, including fruits, vegetables, whole grains, nuts, seeds, and legumes. Each of these components brings its own unique set of flavors and textures to the table. Savoring the natural sweetness of ripe fruits, the crunch of fresh vegetables, the earthy richness of whole grains, and the creamy textures of nuts and seeds not only adds depth to the eating experience but also ensures a broad spectrum of nutrients for optimal health.

The act of savoring flavors and textures goes beyond mere gustatory pleasure; it involves mindfulness and intentional engagement with food. Mindful eating has been linked to various health benefits, including better digestion, improved portion control, and increased satisfaction with meals. For Mind Diet vegans, being attuned to the sensory qualities of their plant-based choices reinforces a positive relationship with food, fostering a sense of gratitude for the nourishment derived from each bite.

Moreover, the mindful savoring of flavors and textures promotes a heightened awareness of satiety signals. By eating slowly and appreciating each mouthful, individuals are more likely to recognize when they are full, reducing the likelihood of overeating. This mindful approach aligns with the Mind Diet's emphasis on portion control and balanced nutritional intake.

In the context of a vegan lifestyle, where creativity in cooking plays a significant role, savoring flavors and textures allows individuals to explore the vast array of culinary possibilities within the plant-based realm. Experimenting with herbs, spices, and various cooking methods becomes a delightful journey of discovery, ensuring that the vegan Mind Diet is not only health-conscious but also an exciting and fulfilling culinary experience.

Savoring flavors and textures is a cornerstone of the Mind Diet for vegans, contributing to both the nutritional richness and psychological satisfaction of the plant-based eating experience.

Continuing the exploration of savoring flavors and textures within the Mind Diet for vegans, it's essential to delve into the broader impact on mental well-being and the potential to foster a positive relationship with food.

1. <u>Mind-Body Connection:</u> Savoring flavors and textures promotes a strong mind-body connection. By being fully present and engaged in the act of eating, individuals can experience a deeper connection to the nourishment they are

providing their bodies. This connection can lead to a heightened sense of overall well-being.

2. <u>Stress Reduction:</u> Mindful savoring has been linked to stress reduction. Taking the time to appreciate the tastes and textures of plant-based meals can create a meditative experience, offering a moment of respite from the demands of daily life. Reduced stress levels contribute positively to cognitive health, aligning with the goals of the Mind Diet.

3. <u>Culinary Creativity:</u> Veganism within the Mind Diet encourages culinary creativity by embracing a wide variety of plant-based ingredients. Savoring flavors and textures becomes an exploration of this diversity, inspiring individuals to experiment with new recipes, herbs, and spices. This creativity not only enhances the pleasure of eating but also adds an element of excitement to the vegan culinary journey.

4. <u>Enhanced Food Appreciation:</u> Mindful savoring cultivates a genuine appreciation for the quality and sourcing of ingredients. Vegans following the Mind Diet often prioritize fresh, locally sourced, and organic produce. By savoring these ingredients, individuals develop a greater awareness of the environmental and

ethical implications of their food choices, contributing to a more sustainable and conscientious approach to eating.

5. <u>Social Connection:</u> Savoring flavors and textures can be a shared experience, fostering social connection and community. Vegan meals prepared with care and enjoyed together create opportunities for bonding over a shared appreciation for wholesome, plant-based foods. This social dimension aligns with the Mind Diet's emphasis on maintaining strong social ties for overall mental well-being.

6. <u>Emotional Satisfaction:</u> Mindful eating acknowledges the emotional aspect of food consumption. Savoring flavors and textures allows individuals to derive emotional satisfaction from their meals, reinforcing positive associations with plant-based choices. This emotional satisfaction contributes to a more positive relationship with food and supports adherence to a vegan Mind Diet over the long term.

In essence, the importance of savoring flavors and textures within the Mind Diet for vegans extends beyond the plate, influencing mental and emotional dimensions. It transforms eating into a holistic experience, where every meal becomes an opportunity for mindfulness, joy, and the cultivation of a positive relationship with

plant-based, nutrient-rich foods.

Chapter 3: Key Nutrients for Cognitive Health

Exploration of nutrients crucial for brain function

Crucial for optimal brain function, several key nutrients play pivotal roles in supporting cognitive health, memory, and overall mental well-being. Here's an extensive overview of these essential nutrients:

1. Omega-3 Fatty Acids:

  - Sources: Fatty fish (salmon, trout, sardines), flaxseeds, chia seeds, walnuts.

  - Role: Omega-3s, particularly EPA and DHA, are fundamental structural components of brain cell membranes. They contribute to neuroplasticity, neurotransmitter function, and have anti-inflammatory properties, protecting against cognitive decline.

2. Antioxidants:

  - Sources: Berries (blueberries, strawberries), dark leafy greens, nuts, seeds, and colorful fruits and vegetables.

  - Role: Antioxidants like vitamins C and E, and phytonutrients such as flavonoids, protect the brain from oxidative stress, neutralizing free radicals that can damage cells and contribute to neurodegenerative diseases.

3. <u>Vitamin B Complex:</u>

  - <u>Sources:</u> Whole grains, legumes, nuts, seeds, leafy greens, avocados.

  - <u>Role:</u> B vitamins, including B6, B9 (folate), and B12, support the production of neurotransmitters, regulate homocysteine levels (elevated levels linked to cognitive decline), and play a crucial role in overall brain health.

4. <u>Vitamin D:</u>

  - <u>Sources:</u> Sunlight exposure, fortified foods (plant-based milk, cereals), mushrooms.

  - <u>Role:</u> Essential for neurodevelopment and function, vitamin D receptors are present in the brain. Adequate levels are associated with a lower risk of cognitive decline.

5. <u>Iron:</u>

  - <u>Sources:</u> Legumes, tofu, nuts, seeds, whole grains, dark leafy greens.

  - <u>Role:</u> Iron is vital for the production of hemoglobin, which transports oxygen to the brain. Iron deficiency can lead to cognitive impairments, affecting memory and concentration.

6. <u>Zinc:</u>

- <u>Sources:</u> Legumes, seeds, nuts, whole grains.

   - <u>Role:</u> Zinc is involved in neurotransmitter function and has antioxidant properties. It supports overall cognitive function and is crucial for learning and memory.

7. <u>Magnesium:</u>

  - <u>Sources:</u> Nuts, seeds, whole grains, leafy greens, legumes.

   - <u>Role:</u> Magnesium participates in synaptic function and is crucial for the activation of many enzymes involved in neurotransmitter synthesis. It plays a role in neuroplasticity and memory.

8. <u>Choline:</u>

  - <u>Sources:</u> Soy products, nuts, seeds, broccoli.

   - <u>Role:</u> Choline is a precursor to acetylcholine, a neurotransmitter involved in memory and mood regulation. Adequate choline intake during pregnancy is crucial for fetal brain development.

9. <u>Protein:</u>

  - <u>Sources:</u> Legumes, tofu, tempeh, seitan, lentils.

- <u>Role:</u> Amino acids from protein sources are essential for neurotransmitter synthesis, supporting communication between brain cells and influencing mood and cognitive function.

10. <u>Fiber:</u>

  - <u>Sources:</u> Whole grains, fruits, vegetables, legumes.

  - <u>Role:</u> While not directly related to brain function, a high-fiber diet supports overall health, including cardiovascular health. A healthy circulatory system ensures adequate blood flow to the brain, supporting cognitive function.

<u>Vegan sources of omega-3 fatty acids, antioxidants, vitamins, and minerals</u>

Here's an overview of vegan sources for omega-3 fatty acids, antioxidants, vitamins, and minerals:

1. <u>Vegan Sources of Omega-3 Fatty Acids:</u>

  - <u>Flaxseeds:</u> Rich in alpha-linolenic acid (ALA), a type of omega-3 fatty acid.

  - <u>Chia Seeds:</u> High in ALA and also provide fiber and protein.

  - <u>Walnuts:</u> Contain ALA and offer additional nutrients like antioxidants and vitamin E.

  - <u>Hemp Seeds:</u> Provide a balanced ratio of omega-3 to omega-6 fatty acids.

2. <u>Vegan Sources of Antioxidants:</u>

- <u>Berries (Blueberries, Strawberries, Raspberries):</u> Packed with anthocyanins and other antioxidants.

- <u>Dark Leafy Greens (Spinach, Kale):</u> Rich in vitamins A, C, and E, as well as various phytonutrients.

- <u>Nuts and Seeds (Almonds, Sunflower Seeds):</u> Provide vitamin E and other antioxidants.

- <u>Colorful Fruits and Vegetables (Bell Peppers, Tomatoes):</u> High in vitamins C and A, and various phytonutrients.

3. <u>Vegan Sources of Vitamins:</u>

- <u>Vitamin C:</u>

- <u>Sources:</u> Citrus fruits (oranges, lemons), strawberries, kiwi, bell peppers, broccoli.

- <u>Vitamin E:</u>

- <u>Sources:</u> Nuts (almonds, hazelnuts), seeds (sunflower seeds, chia seeds), spinach, broccoli.

- <u>Vitamin A (as Beta-Carotene):</u>

- <u>Sources:</u> Carrots, sweet potatoes, butternut squash, kale, spinach.

- <u>Vitamin K:</u>

    - <u>Sources:</u> Leafy greens (kale, spinach, collard greens), broccoli, Brussels sprouts.

4. <u>Vegan Sources of Minerals:</u>

  - <u>Iron:</u>

    - <u>Sources:</u> Legumes (lentils, chickpeas), tofu, quinoa, fortified cereals.

  - <u>Zinc:</u>

    - <u>Sources:</u> Legumes, seeds (pumpkin seeds, hemp seeds), nuts (cashews, almonds), whole grains.

  - <u>Calcium:</u>

    - <u>Sources:</u> Fortified plant milks (soy, almond, oat), tofu, leafy greens (collard greens, kale), almonds.

  - <u>Magnesium:</u>

    - <u>Sources:</u> Nuts (almonds, cashews), seeds (pumpkin seeds, sunflower seeds), whole grains, legumes.

5. <u>Additional Vegan Nutrients:</u>

  - <u>Choline:</u>

    - <u>Sources:</u> Soy products (tofu, tempeh), quinoa, broccoli, Brussels sprouts.

- <u>Protein:</u>

  - <u>Sources:</u> Legumes (beans, lentils), tofu, tempeh, seitan, quinoa.

<u>Chapter 4: Building a Mindful Kitchen</u>

<u>Stocking the pantry with essential vegan ingredients.</u>

Stocking a pantry with essential vegan ingredients is key to maintaining a well-balanced and versatile plant-based diet. Here's a comprehensive list of staples that can form the foundation of a vegan kitchen:

1. <u>Grains and Cereals:</u>

   - Quinoa

   - Brown rice

   - Farro

   - Oats

   - Barley

   - Bulgur

   - Whole wheat pasta

2. <u>Legumes:</u>

   - Lentils (green, brown, red)

   - Chickpeas

   - Black beans

   - Kidney beans

- Cannellini beans

- Pinto beans

3. <u>Protein Sources:</u>

   - Tofu (firm, silken)

   - Tempeh

   - Seitan

   - Edamame

   - Textured vegetable protein (TVP)

4. <u>Nuts and Seeds:</u>

   - Almonds

   - Walnuts

   - Cashews

   - Chia seeds

   - Flaxseeds

   - Sunflower seeds

   - Pumpkin seeds

5. <u>Flour and Baking Essentials:</u>

- All-purpose flour

- Whole wheat flour

- Almond flour

- Baking powder

- Baking soda

- Flaxseed meal (for egg replacement)

6. <u>Herbs and Spices:</u>

- Basil

- Oregano

- Thyme

- Cumin

- Paprika

- Turmeric

- Garlic powder

- Onion powder

- Black pepper

7. <u>Condiments and Sauces:</u>

- Soy sauce or tamari

- Tahini

- Nutritional yeast

- Mustard

- Maple syrup

- Sriracha or hot sauce

- Vegan mayonnaise

- Tomato sauce

8. <u>Plant-Based Milks:</u>

- Almond milk

- Soy milk

- Oat milk

- Coconut milk

9. <u>Whole Fruits and Vegetables:</u>

- Onions

- Garlic

- Potatoes

- Sweet potatoes

- Fresh tomatoes

- Leafy greens (spinach, kale)

10. <u>Frozen Vegetables:</u>

   - Mixed vegetables

   - Peas

   - Corn

   - Broccoli

11. <u>Canned Goods:</u>

   - Canned tomatoes

   - Coconut milk

   - Tomato paste

   - Canned beans (chickpeas, black beans)

12. <u>Whole-Grain Snacks:</u>

   - Whole-grain crackers

   - Brown rice cakes

   - Popcorn kernels

13. <u>Sweeteners:</u>

- Agave syrup

- Maple syrup

- Coconut sugar

14. <u>Healthy Oils:</u>

- Olive oil

- Coconut oil

- Avocado oil

15. <u>Vegan Bouillon or Stock Cubes:</u>

- For quick flavoring of soups and stews.

16. <u>Whole-Grain Pasta and Noodles:</u>

- Whole wheat pasta

- Brown rice noodles

17. <u>Dried Fruits:</u>

- Raisins

- Apricots

- Dates

18. <u>Vegan Chocolate and Cocoa Powder:</u>

   - For baking and sweet treats.

19. <u>Tea and Coffee:</u>

   - Herbal teas

   - Coffee (if desired)

20. <u>Vegan Protein Powders or Shakes:</u>

   - Optional for those looking to supplement protein intake.

Keeping a well-stocked pantry with these essential vegan ingredients ensures a wide variety of options for creating flavorful and nutritious meals. Regularly checking and replenishing supplies can help maintain the flexibility to whip up delicious vegan recipes at any time. Additionally, exploring local markets and specialty stores can introduce new and exciting plant-based ingredients to enhance the culinary experience.

Recommended kitchen tools for a smooth cooking experience

Equipping your kitchen with the right tools can significantly enhance the cooking experience for Mind Diet vegans, making it efficient, enjoyable, and conducive to preparing nutrient-rich meals. Here's a list of recommended kitchen tools:

1. <u>High-Quality Blender:</u>

   - Ideal for creating smoothies, sauces, and creamy soups using a variety of fruits, vegetables, and nuts.

2. <u>Food Processor:</u>

   - Useful for chopping, slicing, and dicing a variety of vegetables, nuts, and seeds. Great for preparing veggie burgers, dips, and energy bites.

3. <u>Vegetable Spiralizer:</u>

   - Perfect for creating vegetable noodles from zucchini, sweet potatoes, or carrots, providing a healthy and gluten-free alternative to pasta.

4. <u>Nut Milk Bag or Cheesecloth:</u>

   - Essential for making homemade nut milks, such as almond or cashew milk.

5. <u>Steamer Basket:</u>

- Ideal for preserving the nutrients in vegetables by gently steaming them. Useful for cooking a variety of greens and other veggies.

6. Mandoline Slicer:

- Allows for precise and uniform slicing of fruits and vegetables, making it easier to create visually appealing dishes and ensuring even cooking.

7. Quality Knives:

- A set of sharp, high-quality knives for chopping, dicing, and slicing various fruits, vegetables, and herbs.

8. Non-Stick Baking Mats or Parchment Paper:

- Perfect for baking without the need for excessive oil, ensuring a healthier cooking process.

9. Instant Pot or Pressure Cooker:

- Speeds up cooking times for grains, legumes, and stews, retaining nutrients while saving time and energy.

10. Silicone Baking Molds:

- Ideal for baking muffins, cupcakes, or energy bars without the need for paper liners or added oils.

11. Citrus Juicer:

   - Effortlessly extracts juice from lemons, limes, and oranges for dressings, marinades, and beverages.

12. Microplane Grater:

   - Useful for zesting citrus fruits, grating ginger, or adding a fine texture to nuts and seeds.

13. High-Speed Blender or Food Processor:

   - Essential for creating smooth nut butters, hummus, and creamy dressings.

14. Vegetable Peeler:

   - Handy for quickly peeling vegetables like carrots and potatoes.

15. Digital Food Scale:

   - Helps with portion control and accurate measurement of ingredients for precise cooking and baking.

16. <u>Non-Stick Cookware:</u>

   - Promotes healthy cooking with minimal oil, making it easier to adhere to the principles of the Mind Diet.

17. <u>Reusable Storage Containers:</u>

   - Ideal for storing prepped ingredients, leftovers, or batch-cooked meals, promoting an organized and sustainable kitchen.

18. <u>Kitchen Timer:</u>

   - Useful for keeping track of cooking times, preventing overcooking or burning.

19. <u>Salad Spinner:</u>

   - Ensures thoroughly dried greens for salads and prevents watery dressings.

20. <u>Herb Mill or Herb Scissors:</u>

   - Facilitates the quick and easy preparation of fresh herbs for added flavor in Mind Diet vegan dishes.

<u>Tips on creating balanced and nutritious vegan meal plans</u>

Creating balanced and nutritious vegan meal plans involves thoughtful consideration of various nutrients to ensure optimal health and well-being. Here are some tips to help you design well-rounded and satisfying vegan meals:

1. <u>Include a Variety of Whole Foods:</u>

   - Incorporate a diverse range of fruits, vegetables, whole grains, legumes, nuts, and seeds to ensure a broad spectrum of essential nutrients.

2. <u>Ensure Protein Adequacy:</u>

   - Include plant-based protein sources such as beans, lentils, tofu, tempeh, quinoa, and edamame to meet protein needs. Combining different protein sources throughout the day can enhance amino acid profiles.

3. <u>Prioritize Whole Grains:</u>

   - Choose whole grains like brown rice, quinoa, oats, and whole wheat to provide fiber, vitamins, and minerals.

4. <u>Incorporate Healthy Fats:</u>

- Include sources of healthy fats such as avocados, nuts, seeds, and olive oil to support brain health and overall well-being.

5. <u>Embrace a Rainbow of Colors:</u>

   - Aim for a colorful plate with a variety of vegetables and fruits. Different colors often indicate different nutrients, providing a well-rounded array of vitamins and antioxidants.

6. <u>Mindful Meal Planning:</u>

   - Plan meals ahead of time to ensure variety and balance. Consider the nutritional content of each meal and spread nutrient-dense foods throughout the day.

7. <u>Don't Forget About B12:</u>

   - Since vitamin B12 is primarily found in animal products, consider fortified foods or supplements to meet B12 needs.

8. <u>Include Iron-Rich Foods:</u>

   - Incorporate iron-rich plant foods such as lentils, beans, tofu, and leafy greens. Consuming vitamin C-rich foods alongside iron sources enhances absorption.

9. Calcium-Rich Choices:

   - Ensure adequate calcium intake through fortified plant milks, tofu, leafy greens (kale, bok choy), and fortified orange juice.

10. Hydration is Key:

   - Drink plenty of water throughout the day to stay hydrated. Consider herbal teas or infused water for added variety.

11. Watch Portion Sizes:

   - Be mindful of portion sizes to maintain a healthy weight and prevent overeating.

12. Experiment with Herbs and Spices:

   - Enhance flavors without added salt or excessive oil by using a variety of herbs and spices. This not only adds taste but also provides additional health benefits.

13. Be Cautious with Processed Foods:

   - Limit processed and refined foods. While convenient, they can be high in added sugars, salt, and unhealthy fats.

14. <u>Include Omega-3 Fatty Acids:</u>

   - Ensure an adequate intake of omega-3 fatty acids through sources like flaxseeds, chia seeds, walnuts, and algae-based supplements.

15. <u>Consider Nutrient Timing:</u>

   - Distribute nutrients strategically throughout the day. For example, consider having a source of protein in each meal and snacks to support muscle maintenance and satiety.

16. <u>Listen to Your Body:</u>

   - Pay attention to hunger and fullness cues. Eating intuitively helps maintain a healthy relationship with food.

17. <u>Seek Professional Guidance:</u>

   - Consult with a registered dietitian or nutritionist for personalized advice, especially if you have specific dietary requirements or health concerns.

<u>Incorporating variety and color in meals for optimal health</u>

Incorporating variety and color into meals is a fundamental principle of the Mind Diet for vegans, promoting optimal health by ensuring a diverse array of nutrients. Here's why and how to embrace variety and color in your vegan meals:

1. <u>Nutrient Diversity:</u>

   - Different colored fruits and vegetables often indicate distinct sets of vitamins, minerals, and antioxidants. By consuming a variety, you maximize your intake of essential nutrients, supporting overall well-being.

2. <u>Phytonutrient Richness:</u>

   - The pigments responsible for vibrant colors in plant foods are often phytonutrients with potential health benefits. These compounds can have antioxidant, anti-inflammatory, and immune-boosting properties.

3. <u>Balanced Nutrient Intake:</u>

   - Different plant foods provide varying nutrient profiles. Including a spectrum of colors ensures a balanced intake of carbohydrates, proteins, healthy fats, vitamins, and minerals.

4. <u>Eye-Catching Appeal:</u>

- A visually appealing plate is more enjoyable to eat. Colorful meals stimulate the senses, making the dining experience more satisfying and promoting a positive relationship with food.

5. Mood and Mental Well-Being:

- The diversity of nutrients in colorful plant foods can contribute to mental well-being. For instance, foods rich in omega-3 fatty acids (found in walnuts, chia seeds, and flaxseeds) have been linked to improved mood and cognitive function.

6. Meal Satisfaction and Satiation:

- A variety of colors often means a variety of textures and flavors. This sensory diversity can enhance satisfaction, making you feel more satiated after meals.

7. Easy Implementation:

- Incorporating variety and color doesn't have to be complicated. A simple strategy is to aim for a "rainbow" on your plate, including fruits and vegetables of different colors in each meal.

8. Seasonal Eating:

- Embrace seasonal produce for both freshness and optimal nutrient content. Seasonal fruits and vegetables often offer a richer nutritional profile.

9. Meal Planning and Prepping:

- Plan meals that include a mix of colorful ingredients. When prepping, chop a variety of vegetables to have on hand for quick and easy additions to meals.

10. Creative Cooking Methods:

- Experiment with different cooking methods to preserve colors and flavors. Lightly steaming or roasting vegetables can enhance their natural vibrancy.

11. Colorful Salads:

- Create salads with a mix of greens, colorful vegetables, fruits, and nuts. Adding a variety of textures and flavors makes salads more enjoyable and nutritious.

12. Smoothie Bowls:

- Blend vibrant fruits and vegetables into smoothie bowls. Top them with nuts, seeds, and colorful berries for added variety and nutrition.

13. <u>Diverse Grain Bowls:</u>

- Build grain bowls with a combination of colorful vegetables, legumes, and whole grains. Consider using quinoa, brown rice, or farro as a base.

14. <u>Fruit-Based Desserts:</u>

- Opt for fruit-based desserts like fruit salads, grilled fruit, or fruit sorbets to satisfy sweet cravings while adding a burst of color.

15. <u>Explore Exotic Ingredients:</u>

- Experiment with less familiar, colorful, and nutrient-rich ingredients like dragon fruit, purple sweet potatoes, or watermelon radishes for culinary diversity.

Chapter 6: Mind Diet Vegan Recipes

Breakfast options promoting mental clarity

Promoting mental clarity through a Mind Diet vegan breakfast involves incorporating nutrient-dense foods that support cognitive function and overall brain health. Here are some breakfast options that align with the Mind Diet principles:

1. Berry Smoothie Bowl:

   - Blend a mix of berries (blueberries, strawberries, raspberries) with a banana and plant-based yogurt. Top with granola, chia seeds, and a sprinkle of nuts for added texture and omega-3 fatty acids.

2. Avocado Toast with Whole Grain Bread:

   - Spread mashed avocado on whole-grain toast. Top with sliced tomatoes, a sprinkle of chia seeds, and a dash of lemon juice. Avocado provides healthy fats, while whole grains offer complex carbohydrates for sustained energy.

3. Chia Seed Pudding:

   - Mix chia seeds with your favorite plant-based milk and let it sit overnight. In the morning, top with fresh fruits, such as kiwi and pomegranate seeds, for a nutrient-rich and satisfying pudding.

4. <u>Oatmeal with Nuts and Berries:</u>

   - Cook steel-cut oats with plant-based milk and top with a variety of nuts (almonds, walnuts) and berries. Oats contain beta-glucans, supporting heart health and providing a steady release of energy.

5. <u>Tofu Scramble:</u>

   - Sauté tofu with colorful vegetables like bell peppers, spinach, and tomatoes. Season with turmeric, black salt, and pepper for a flavorful and protein-packed breakfast.

6. <u>Quinoa Breakfast Bowl:</u>

   - Cook quinoa and top it with sliced banana, diced mango, and a handful of nuts. Drizzle with almond butter or tahini for added richness and healthy fats.

7. <u>Vegan Breakfast Burrito:</u>

   - Fill a whole-grain tortilla with black beans, sautéed vegetables, avocado, and salsa. The combination provides a balance of protein, fiber, and healthy fats.

8. <u>L-Plant-Based Yogurt Parfait:</u>

- Layer plant-based yogurt with granola, mixed berries, and a sprinkle of seeds like flaxseeds or pumpkin seeds. This parfait offers a blend of textures and nutrients.

9. <u>Sweet Potato and Chickpea Hash:</u>

   - Sauté sweet potatoes and chickpeas with onions and spices like cumin and paprika. Top with avocado slices and fresh herbs for a savory and nutrient-rich breakfast.

10. <u>Green Smoothie:</u>

   - Blend a mix of leafy greens (kale, spinach), a banana, and pineapple for a refreshing green smoothie. Add chia seeds or hemp seeds for an extra boost of omega-3s.

11. <u>Nut Butter Banana Toast:</u>

   - Spread almond or peanut butter on whole-grain toast and top with banana slices. Nut butters provide healthy fats, while bananas offer natural sweetness and potassium.

12. <u>Vegan Pancakes or Waffles:</u>

- Prepare pancakes or waffles using whole-grain flour or a mix of flours like almond and oat. Top with fresh fruit, such as berries or sliced peaches, and a dollop of plant-based yogurt.

<u>Lunch and dinner recipes rich in brain-boosting nutrients</u>

Creating lunch and dinner recipes rich in brain-boosting nutrients for Mind Diet vegans involves incorporating a variety of colorful, nutrient-dense ingredients. Here are some delicious and brain-nourishing recipes:

<u>Lunch Options:</u>

1. <u>Quinoa Salad with Chickpeas and Vegetables:</u>

   - Toss cooked quinoa with chickpeas, cherry tomatoes, cucumber, and bell peppers. Dress with olive oil, lemon juice, and fresh herbs like parsley. Top with a sprinkle of pumpkin seeds for added crunch and zinc.

2. <u>Stuffed Bell Peppers with Lentils and Spinach:</u>

   - Roast bell peppers and fill them with a mixture of cooked lentils, spinach, tomatoes, and spices. Bake until peppers are tender and serve with a side of quinoa.

3. Vegan Mediterranean Wrap:

- Fill a whole-grain wrap with hummus, sliced cucumber, cherry tomatoes, olives, and fresh herbs. Add a drizzle of extra virgin olive oil for healthy fats.

4. Sweet Potato and Black Bean Bowl:

- Roast sweet potatoes and toss with black beans, corn, and diced avocado. Sprinkle with cumin and coriander for flavor, and serve over brown rice.

Dinner Options:

1. Lemon Garlic Herb Baked Tofu:

- Marinate tofu cubes in a mixture of lemon juice, garlic, and herbs. Bake until golden brown and serve over a bed of quinoa or with sautéed greens.

2. Chickpea and Vegetable Stir-Fry:

- Sauté chickpeas, broccoli, carrots, and bell peppers in a flavorful stir-fry sauce made with soy sauce, ginger, and garlic. Serve over brown rice or noodles.

3. Curried Lentil and Vegetable Stew:

- Simmer lentils with a medley of colorful vegetables in a rich curry broth. Add turmeric for an anti-inflammatory boost and serve over couscous or quinoa.

4. <u>Cauliflower and Chickpea Curry:</u>

  - Cook cauliflower and chickpeas in a coconut milk-based curry sauce with spices like cumin, coriander, and turmeric. Serve over basmati rice.

<u>Sides and Extras:</u>

1. <u>Garlic Roasted Brussels Sprouts:</u>

  - Roast Brussels sprouts with garlic, olive oil, and a pinch of sea salt. These provide vitamin K and antioxidants.

2. <u>Kale and Walnut Pesto Pasta:</u>

  - Blend kale, walnuts, nutritional yeast, garlic, and olive oil to create a vibrant pesto. Toss with whole-grain pasta for a brain-boosting dish.

3. <u>Turmeric Roasted Carrots:</u>

  - Roast carrots with turmeric, black pepper, and a touch of maple syrup. Turmeric contains curcumin, known for its anti-inflammatory properties.

<u>**Snacks and desserts with a focus on cognitive well-being**</u>

Creating snacks and desserts that prioritize cognitive well-being for Mind Diet vegans involves incorporating nutrient-dense ingredients known for their brain-boosting properties. Here are some delicious and mindful recipes:

<u>Snacks:</u>

1. <u>Trail Mix with Nuts and Berries:</u>

   - Mix almonds, walnuts, pumpkin seeds, and dried berries. Nuts provide healthy fats, while berries offer antioxidants.

2. <u>Guacamole with Veggie Sticks:</u>

   - Mash avocado with lime juice, garlic, and cilantro. Serve with carrot and cucumber sticks for a satisfying snack rich in healthy fats.

3. <u>Roasted Chickpeas:</u>

   - Toss chickpeas with olive oil and spices like cumin and paprika. Roast until crunchy for a protein-packed snack with fiber.

4. Edamame Hummus with Whole Grain Crackers:

   - Blend edamame with tahini, lemon juice, and garlic to create a vibrant hummus. Pair with whole-grain crackers for a tasty and nourishing snack.

Desserts:

1. Blueberry Chia Seed Pudding:

   - Mix chia seeds with almond milk and let it set. Layer with blueberry compote and top with fresh blueberries. Chia seeds offer omega-3 fatty acids.

2. Dark Chocolate Avocado Mousse:

   - Blend ripe avocado, dark chocolate, and a touch of maple syrup. Chill and enjoy a decadent mousse rich in healthy fats and antioxidants.

3. Baked Apple Slices with Cinnamon:

   - Slice apples and toss with cinnamon. Bake until tender for a naturally sweet treat with added antioxidants.

4. Turmeric Golden Milk Popsicles:

- Mix coconut milk with turmeric, ginger, and a hint of black pepper. Freeze into popsicles for a refreshing and anti-inflammatory dessert.

Energy Bites:

1. Almond Butter Energy Balls:

   - Combine almond butter, oats, chia seeds, and a drizzle of agave syrup. Roll into bite-sized balls for a convenient and energy-boosting snack.

2. Matcha Bliss Balls:

   - Blend dates, almonds, and matcha powder. Roll into balls and coat with shredded coconut. Matcha provides a gentle caffeine boost.

3. Walnut and Fig Bars:

   - Blend walnuts, dried figs, and a pinch of cinnamon. Press into a pan and chill for a delicious, no-bake snack with omega-3 fatty acids.

Drinks:

1. Berry and Spinach Smoothie:

- Blend mixed berries, spinach, banana, and plant-based yogurt. The combination offers vitamins, antioxidants, and a refreshing flavor.

2. <u>Turmeric Latte with Almond Milk:</u>

- Heat almond milk with turmeric, ginger, and a touch of maple syrup. This warming drink combines anti-inflammatory ingredients.

<u>Vegan alternatives for classic dishes with a mindful twist</u>

Creating vegan alternatives for classic dishes with a mindful twist involves incorporating plant-based ingredients while maintaining the essence and flavors of the original recipes. Here are some thoughtful and delicious vegan adaptations:

1. <u>Vegan Spaghetti Bolognese:</u>

   - Substitute ground meat with lentils or finely chopped mushrooms for a hearty and protein-packed version. Add tomatoes, garlic, onions, and herbs for the traditional Bolognese flavor.

2. <u>Vegan Tacos with Walnut "Meat":</u>

   - Pulse walnuts, black beans, and spices in a food processor to create a savory and textured walnut "meat" for taco filling. Top with guacamole, salsa, and fresh cilantro.

3. <u>Chickpea and Vegetable Curry:</u>

   - Replace meat with chickpeas in classic curry recipes. Load it with colorful vegetables, coconut milk, and a blend of spices for a flavorful and nutrient-dense alternative.

4. <u>Vegan Caesar Salad:</u>

- Make a creamy Caesar dressing using cashews, nutritional yeast, garlic, and lemon juice. Toss it with crisp romaine lettuce, croutons, and vegan parmesan for a plant-powered Caesar salad.

5. <u>Vegan Pizza with Cashew Cheese:</u>

- Create a dairy-free cashew cheese by blending soaked cashews with nutritional yeast and herbs. Use it as a topping on a pizza loaded with fresh veggies for a mindful twist on a classic.

6. <u>Eggplant Lasagna:</u>

- Replace traditional lasagna noodles with thinly sliced and grilled eggplant layers. Alternate them with vegan ricotta, marinara sauce, and spinach for a lighter and plant-centric lasagna.

7. <u>Vegan Burger with Portobello Mushroom Patty:</u>

- Grill or roast portobello mushrooms as the burger patty. Top with lettuce, tomato, avocado, and vegan mayo for a satisfying and umami-rich burger.

8. Vegan Pad Thai with Tofu:

   - Swap out shrimp or chicken for tofu in Pad Thai. Toss with rice noodles, bean sprouts, peanuts, and a flavorful tamarind-based sauce for a vegan-friendly version.

9. Vegan Mac and "Cheese" with Butternut Squash Sauce:

   - Puree roasted butternut squash with nutritional yeast, garlic, and plant-based milk for a creamy "cheese" sauce. Pour it over whole-grain pasta for a comforting and nutritious mac and cheese.

10. Cauliflower Buffalo Wings:

   - Coat cauliflower florets in a batter and bake until crispy. Toss them in buffalo sauce for a spicy and satisfying alternative to traditional chicken wings.

11. Vegan Sushi with Avocado and Vegetable Rolls:

   - Fill sushi rolls with avocado, cucumber, carrots, and other colorful vegetables. Serve with soy sauce and wasabi for a mindful and plant-based sushi experience.

12. Vegan Chocolate Avocado Mousse:

   - Blend ripe avocados with cocoa powder, maple syrup, and vanilla for a rich and creamy chocolate mousse. Chill and enjoy a decadent dessert without dairy.

Substituting animal products without compromising flavor

Substituting animal products in Mind Diet vegan recipes without compromising flavor involves choosing plant-based alternatives that bring rich tastes and textures to the dish. Here are some thoughtful substitutions to maintain deliciousness while adhering to Mind Diet principles:

1. Plant-Based Proteins:

   - Substitute for Ground Meat: Use lentils, mushrooms, or a mix of grains and legumes for a hearty and flavorful replacement in dishes like chili, tacos, or Bolognese.

   - Substitute for Chicken: Utilize tofu, tempeh, or seitan for a versatile and protein-packed alternative in stir-fries, curries, or sandwiches.

   - Substitute for Fish: Try marinated and grilled tofu or heart of palm for a satisfying texture in dishes like fish tacos or vegan fish and chips.

2. Dairy Alternatives:

   - Milk Substitute: Opt for almond, soy, or oat milk in recipes calling for dairy milk. Choose unsweetened varieties for savory dishes to maintain the intended flavor.

- <u>Cheese Substitute:</u> Use nut-based cheeses or nutritional yeast to add a cheesy and savory element to dishes. Vegan mozzarella or cashew-based spreads work well in pizzas and pastas.

3. <u>Egg Replacements:</u>

- <u>For Binding:</u> Mix flaxseeds or chia seeds with water to create a gel-like consistency, serving as an excellent egg substitute in baking.

- <u>For Leavening:</u> Blend mashed bananas, applesauce, or vinegar with baking soda to replicate the leavening effects of eggs in baked goods.

4. <u>Butter Alternatives:</u>

- <u>Cooking and Baking:</u> Substitute olive oil, coconut oil, or vegan margarine in equal proportions for a rich and flavorful option in both savory and sweet dishes.

5. <u>Umami Boosters:</u>

- <u>Mushrooms:</u> Finely chop or blend mushrooms to add a meaty and umami flavor to dishes like burgers, stews, or risottos.

- <u>Tamari or Soy Sauce:</u> Use these for a depth of flavor and savory richness in place of traditional soy sauce.

6. <u>Flavorful Herbs and Spices:</u>

   - <u>Fresh Herbs:</u> Enhance flavors with fresh herbs like basil, cilantro, mint, or dill to bring brightness and complexity to various dishes.

   - <u>Spices:</u> Experiment with spices such as cumin, smoked paprika, coriander, and turmeric to add depth and warmth to your meals.

7. <u>Nuts and Seeds for Texture:</u>

   - <u>Crunchy Toppings:</u> Add chopped nuts (like almonds or walnuts) or seeds (like pumpkin or sunflower seeds) to salads, stir-fries, or grain bowls for a satisfying crunch.

8. <u>Mindful Cooking Techniques:</u>

   - <u>Grilling and Roasting:</u> These methods enhance flavors and textures, especially when applied to vegetables, tofu, or plant-based proteins.

   - <u>Sautéing:</u> Use a variety of vegetables, garlic, and onions to create a flavorful base for many dishes.

9. <u>Mindful Seasoning:</u>

- <u>Low-Sodium Options:</u> Be mindful of salt intake by incorporating herbs, spices, and citrus for seasoning. Freshly ground black pepper can add a punch without excessive sodium.

Chapter 8: Mindful Eating Habits

Portion control and mindful serving sizes

Portion control and mindful serving sizes play a crucial role in adhering to the principles of the Mind Diet for vegans, promoting optimal health and cognitive well-being. Here are some tips for managing portions and serving sizes mindfully:

1. Balance Macronutrients:

   - Aim for a balanced distribution of macronutrients in each meal. Include a source of plant-based protein, whole grains, healthy fats, and a variety of colorful vegetables. This not only supports satiety but also provides a diverse range of nutrients.

2. Listen to Hunger Cues:

   - Pay attention to your body's hunger and fullness signals. Eat when you're hungry and stop when you're satisfied. Practice mindful eating by savoring each bite and being present during meals.

3. Use Smaller Plates and Bowls:

- Opt for smaller dinnerware to visually trick the mind into perceiving larger portions. This can help prevent overeating and promote a sense of satisfaction with smaller servings.

4. <u>Start with Smaller Portions:</u>

- Begin with smaller portions, especially when trying new recipes or dishes. You can always go back for more if you're still hungry, but starting with a smaller serving encourages mindfulness.

5. <u>Include a Variety of Foods:</u>

- Create a colorful and diverse plate by incorporating a variety of fruits, vegetables, legumes, whole grains, and plant-based proteins. This not only enhances nutritional intake but also adds visual appeal to meals.

6. <u>Practice Mindful Snacking:</u>

- When snacking, portion out a serving rather than eating directly from the package. This helps prevent mindless overeating and allows you to be more aware of the quantity consumed.

7. <u>Be Aware of Liquid Calories:</u>

- Mindfully consume beverages, including plant-based smoothies, juices, and nut milks. While these can be nutritious, liquid calories can add up quickly. Consider measuring servings and being conscious of added sugars.

8. <u>Use Measuring Tools:</u>

   - Initially, use measuring cups or a food scale to gauge proper portion sizes. This can help develop a better understanding of what constitutes a serving and contribute to more accurate portion control.

9. <u>Plate Half-Full of Vegetables:</u>

   - Fill half of your plate with a variety of colorful vegetables. Vegetables are nutrient-dense and low in calories, making them a great foundation for a well-balanced and satisfying meal.

10. <u>Mindful Eating Practices:</u>

   - Chew your food thoroughly and savor each bite. Eating slowly allows your body to recognize when it's full, preventing overeating.

11. <u>Understand Serving Size Recommendations:</u>

- Familiarize yourself with recommended serving sizes for different food groups. This knowledge can guide you in creating balanced and appropriately sized meals.

12. <u>Be Conscious of Energy Density:</u>

- Choose foods with lower energy density, meaning they have fewer calories per gram. These foods, often high in fiber and water content, can be more filling and supportive of weight management.

13. <u>Plan and Prepare Meals in Advance:</u>

- Preparing meals in advance allows you to control portion sizes more effectively. Portion out meals into containers for easy access, especially during busy days.

14. <u>Enjoy Treats in Moderation:</u>

- While treats and indulgences can be part of a balanced diet, consume them in moderation. Be mindful of portion sizes, and savor these treats as occasional delights rather than regular indulgences.

<u>The importance of savoring each bite and eating without distractions</u>

Savoring each bite and practicing mindful eating without distractions are essential components of the Mind Diet for vegans, fostering a deeper connection with food and promoting overall well-being. Here's why these practices are important:

1. <u>Enhances Sensory Experience:</u>

   - Savoring each bite allows you to fully engage your senses. Appreciate the colors, textures, aromas, and flavors of your food, creating a more gratifying and enjoyable eating experience.

2. <u>Promotes Digestive Health:</u>

   - Mindful eating encourages thorough chewing, breaking down food into smaller particles. This aids in the digestion process, making it easier for the body to absorb nutrients and support optimal digestive health.

3. <u>Recognizes Hunger and Fullness:</u>

   - Eating without distractions enables you to tune into your body's hunger and fullness cues. By being present during meals, you are more likely to eat in response to actual physical hunger rather than external triggers.

4. <u>Prevents Overeating:</u>

- Distractions like TV, phones, or computers can lead to mindless eating, where you consume larger portions without realizing it. Focusing on your meal helps prevent overeating by allowing you to register the feeling of fullness more accurately.

5. Cultivates Gratitude:

   - Mindful eating fosters a sense of gratitude for the nourishment your food provides. By savoring each bite, you develop a deeper appreciation for the effort involved in growing, preparing, and bringing food to your table.

6. Promotes Mind-Body Connection:

   - Being fully present during meals nurtures a stronger mind-body connection. Understanding how different foods make you feel can guide food choices that align with your overall well-being.

7. Reduces Stress and Anxiety:

   - Eating without distractions allows you to focus on the present moment, reducing stress and anxiety associated with external pressures. It creates a peaceful and mindful atmosphere around mealtime.

8. <u>Encourages Intuitive Eating:</u>

- Mindful eating supports the practice of intuitive eating, where you trust your body's signals for hunger and fullness. This fosters a healthier relationship with food and a more intuitive approach to nourishing your body.

9. <u>Enhances Enjoyment and Satisfaction:</u>

- Taking the time to savor each bite increases the pleasure derived from your meals. This heightened enjoyment can lead to greater satisfaction and a more positive attitude toward the foods you consume.

10. <u>Aids in Weight Management:</u>

- By paying attention to your food and eating slowly, you allow your body to recognize when it's satisfied. This can contribute to better portion control and support weight management goals.

11. <u>Fosters Mindful Food Choices:</u>

- When you eat without distractions, you are more likely to make intentional and mindful food choices. This can lead to selecting nutrient-dense, whole foods that align with the principles of the Mind Diet.

12. <u>Cultivates a Sense of Ritual:</u>

- Eating mindfully can transform mealtime into a ritual. This intentional practice brings a sense of purpose and mindfulness to nourishing your body, fostering a positive relationship with food.

<u>Chapter 9: Culinary Techniques for Flavorful Vegan Dishes:</u>

<u>Cooking methods to enhance flavors without excessive use of oils or processed</u>

<u>ingredients</u>

Cooking methods that enhance flavors without relying on excessive oils or processed ingredients align with the mindful and health-conscious principles of the Mind Diet for vegans. Here are cooking techniques that bring out robust flavors while prioritizing whole, plant-based foods:

1. <u>Grilling and Roasting:</u>

   - <u>Technique:</u> Grilling or roasting vegetables intensifies their natural sweetness and adds a smoky flavor.

   - Tips: Brush vegetables lightly with olive oil or a marinade made from herbs, spices, and citrus for enhanced flavor without excessive oil.

2. <u>Sautéing with Vegetable Broth or Water:</u>

   - <u>Technique:</u> Sautéing with vegetable broth or water instead of oil adds flavor while reducing fat content.

   - <u>Tips:</u> Use flavorful ingredients like garlic, onions, and herbs to create a fragrant base for sautéed dishes.

3. Steam-Baking:

  - Technique: Steam-baking involves using a small amount of water to create steam while baking, keeping dishes moist without excess oil.

  - Tips: Steam-bake vegetables or grains by adding a layer of water to the baking dish and covering it with foil.

4. Marinating with Herbs and Spices:

  - Technique: Marinating tofu, tempeh, or vegetables in a mixture of herbs, spices, and acidic ingredients enhances flavor without relying on processed sauces.

  - Tips: Combine ingredients like garlic, ginger, lemon juice, and a variety of herbs for a flavorful marinade.

5. Stir-Frying with Tamari or Soy Sauce:

  - Technique: Stir-frying with minimal oil and using tamari or soy sauce adds savory depth to the dish.

  - Tips: Incorporate colorful vegetables, tofu, or tempeh for a quick and flavorful stir-fry.

6. Herb and Spice Rubs:

- <u>Technique:</u> Creating herb and spice rubs for roasted or grilled vegetables intensifies their taste.

- <u>Tips:</u> Mix herbs like rosemary, thyme, and oregano with spices such as cumin and paprika to create versatile rubs.

7. Slow Cooking:

- <u>Technique:</u> Slow cooking allows flavors to meld, resulting in rich and hearty plant-based dishes.

- <u>Tips:</u> Utilize a variety of beans, lentils, vegetables, and aromatic herbs to create flavorful stews and soups.

8. Vinegar and Citrus Zest:

- <u>Technique:</u> Incorporate balsamic vinegar, apple cider vinegar, or citrus zest to add brightness and tang to dishes.

- <u>Tips:</u> Use these ingredients in dressings, marinades, or as a finishing touch to enhance flavors.

9. Smoking with Natural Wood Chips:

- <u>Technique:</u> Smoking vegetables or plant-based proteins using natural wood chips imparts a smoky flavor without added oils.

- <u>Tips:</u> Experiment with different types of wood chips, such as hickory or mesquite, to add depth to the smokiness.

10. <u>Tomato-Based Sauces:</u>

   - <u>Technique:</u> Creating tomato-based sauces with fresh or canned tomatoes adds richness and depth to pasta dishes, stews, and casseroles.

   - <u>Tips:</u> Enhance sauces with garlic, onions, and a variety of herbs for robust flavors.

11. <u>Herb-Infused Broths:</u>

   - <u>Technique:</u> Infuse broths with fresh herbs and aromatic vegetables for a flavorful base in soups, stews, and grain dishes.

   - <u>Tips:</u> Simmer a mix of herbs like parsley, thyme, and bay leaves with vegetables like onions and carrots to create a fragrant broth.

12. <u>Herb Garnishes:</u>

   - <u>Technique:</u> Garnish dishes with fresh herbs like basil, cilantro, or mint just before serving to add a burst of flavor.

   - <u>Tips:</u> Keep a selection of fresh herbs on hand to elevate the taste of meals without added calories.

Techniques for maximizing the nutritional value of ingredients

Maximizing the nutritional value of ingredients is a key aspect of the Mind Diet for vegans, aiming to support cognitive health through nutrient-rich and diverse plant-based foods. Here are techniques to enhance the nutritional content of ingredients:

1. Include a Variety of Colorful Vegetables:

- Technique: Incorporate a diverse array of colorful vegetables to ensure a wide range of vitamins, minerals, and antioxidants.

- Tips: Aim for a rainbow on your plate, including dark leafy greens, vibrant bell peppers, carrots, beets, and tomatoes.

2. Choose Whole Grains:

- Technique: Opt for whole grains over refined grains to maximize fiber content and retain essential nutrients.

- Tips: Choose quinoa, brown rice, barley, farro, and whole wheat products to increase fiber, vitamins, and minerals.

3. Prioritize Plant-Based Proteins:

- Technique: Select a variety of plant-based protein sources such as legumes, tofu, tempeh, and edamame to ensure a well-rounded amino acid profile.

- Tips: Experiment with different beans, lentils, and ancient grains like quinoa and amaranth for diverse plant-based protein options.

4. Incorporate Nuts and Seeds:

- Technique: Include a mix of nuts and seeds to provide healthy fats, protein, and essential micronutrients.

- Tips: Sprinkle chia seeds, flaxseeds, almonds, walnuts, and pumpkin seeds onto salads, yogurt, or smoothie bowls for added nutrition.

5. Embrace Healthy Fats:

- Technique: Choose sources of healthy fats such as avocados, olives, nuts, and seeds to support brain health and enhance absorption of fat-soluble vitamins.

- Tips: Use avocados in sandwiches, salads, or as a creamy base for sauces and dressings.

6. Experiment with Seaweed and Algae:

- Technique: Incorporate seaweed and algae for plant-based sources of omega-3 fatty acids, vitamins, and minerals.

- <u>Tips:</u> Add nori to salads, use spirulina in smoothies, or experiment with dishes featuring kelp or dulse.

7. <u>Include a Variety of Fruits:</u>

- <u>Technique:</u> Integrate a diverse range of fruits to obtain a spectrum of vitamins, antioxidants, and natural sugars.

- <u>Tips:</u> Mix seasonal fruits in salads, enjoy them as snacks, or blend them into smoothies for a burst of flavor and nutrition.

8. <u>Use Fresh Herbs and Spices:</u>

- <u>Technique:</u> Enhance flavors without excessive salt or processed seasonings by using fresh herbs and spices.

- <u>Tips:</u> Experiment with basil, cilantro, parsley, turmeric, cumin, and other herbs and spices to add depth and nutritional benefits.

9. <u>Opt for Fermented Foods:</u>

- <u>Technique:</u> Incorporate fermented foods like sauerkraut, kimchi, tempeh, and miso for gut health and increased nutrient absorption.

- <u>Tips:</u> Include a small serving of fermented foods as a side or condiment to diversify your microbiome.

10. <u>Choose Seasonal and Local Produce:</u>

- Technique: Prioritize seasonal and local produce for maximum freshness and nutritional value.

- <u>Tips:</u> Visit farmers' markets or join a community-supported agriculture (CSA) program to access locally grown, nutrient-rich ingredients.

11. <u>Steam or Roast Vegetables Lightly:</u>

- <u>Technique:</u> Steam or lightly roast vegetables to retain their nutrients while enhancing flavor.

- <u>Tips:</u> Use minimal oil and season with herbs and spices to preserve the nutritional content of vegetables.

12. <u>Prepare Balanced and Diverse Meals:</u>

- <u>Technique:</u> Create meals with a balance of carbohydrates, proteins, and fats, using a variety of plant-based ingredients.

- <u>Tips:</u> Combine grains, legumes, vegetables, and healthy fats in diverse ways to ensure a comprehensive nutritional profile in each meal.

<u>**Chapter 10: Seasonal and Local Ingredients**</u>

<u>**Highlighting the benefits of using seasonal and locally sourced produce**</u>

Using seasonal and locally sourced produce aligns seamlessly with the Mind Diet for vegans, offering a multitude of benefits that contribute to both cognitive health and overall well-being. Here are the key advantages of incorporating seasonal and locally sourced produce into a Mind Diet vegan lifestyle:

1. <u>Enhanced Nutrient Content:</u>

   - <u>Benefit:</u> Seasonal produce is often harvested at its peak ripeness, providing optimal nutrient content. Locally sourced items have shorter transportation times, minimizing nutrient loss.

   - <u>Impact:</u> Higher nutrient levels contribute to better cognitive health, supporting the Mind Diet's emphasis on foods rich in vitamins, minerals, and antioxidants.

2. <u>Improved Flavor and Texture:</u>

   - <u>Benefit:</u> Seasonal produce tends to be fresher, delivering superior taste and texture. Locally sourced items are harvested closer to the time of purchase, ensuring a more enjoyable culinary experience.

   - <u>Impact:</u> Enhanced flavor and texture encourage mindful eating, promoting satisfaction and pleasure from plant-based meals.

3. <u>Support for Local Agriculture:</u>

- <u>Benefit:</u> Choosing locally sourced produce supports local farmers and agriculture. This, in turn, fosters a sense of community and strengthens regional food systems.

- <u>Impact:</u> Aligning with the Mind Diet involves not only personal well-being but also contributing to sustainable and resilient food practices within local communities.

4. <u>Reduced Environmental Impact:</u>

- <u>Benefit:</u> Seasonal and local produce often requires less energy for transportation and storage, leading to a lower carbon footprint.

- <u>Impact:</u> Aligning with Mind Diet principles emphasizes holistic well-being, and reducing environmental impact supports broader ecological health, creating a harmonious relationship between personal and planetary well-being.

5. <u>Diverse and Varied Diet:</u>

- <u>Benefit:</u> Seasonal availability encourages variety in the diet, exposing individuals to a broader range of nutrients and phytochemicals. Local sourcing introduces unique and indigenous varieties of fruits and vegetables.

- <u>Impact:</u> A diverse and varied diet, in line with the Mind Diet, ensures a spectrum of nutrients beneficial for cognitive health and overall nutritional balance.

6. <u>Seasonal Eating Aligns with Nature's Cycles:</u>

   - <u>Benefit:</u> Consuming seasonal produce aligns with the natural cycles of the environment, providing the nutrients our bodies need during different times of the year.

   - <u>Impact:</u> This practice resonates with the Mind Diet's holistic approach, recognizing the interconnectedness of personal health with the natural world.

7. <u>Affordability and Cost Savings:</u>

   - <u>Benefit:</u> Seasonal produce is often more abundant and less expensive due to local abundance and reduced transportation costs.

   - <u>Impact:</u> Affordability promotes accessibility to fresh, nutritious foods, making a Mind Diet approach more inclusive and sustainable for a wider range of individuals.

8. <u>Increased Awareness of Food Origins:</u>

- <u>Benefit:</u> Choosing locally sourced produce fosters awareness of where food comes from, promoting transparency and a deeper connection with the source of one's nutrition.

- <u>Impact:</u> Mindful eating involves not only the consumption of food but also an understanding and appreciation of its origins, creating a more conscious and intentional relationship with the act of nourishment.

9. <u>Encourages Seasonal Meal Planning:</u>

- <u>Benefit:</u> Seasonal and local sourcing inspires creativity in meal planning, encouraging individuals to adapt recipes based on what is readily available.

- <u>Impact:</u> This adaptability aligns with the Mind Diet's emphasis on flexibility and variety in food choices, promoting a dynamic and sustainable approach to plant-based eating.

<u>Connecting with the environment and supporting sustainable practices</u>

Connecting with the environment and supporting sustainable practices is a holistic aspect of the Mind Diet for vegans, reflecting a broader commitment to well-being that extends beyond personal health. Here are the ways in which embracing sustainable practices aligns with the principles of the Mind Diet for a more mindful and environmentally conscious lifestyle:

1. <u>Local and Seasonal Eating:</u>

   - <u>Connection with Environment:</u> Choosing locally sourced and seasonal produce fosters a direct connection with the local environment, as it aligns with the natural cycles and availability of foods in the region.

   - <u>Sustainable Impact:</u> By supporting local farmers and reducing the carbon footprint associated with transportation, individuals contribute to a more sustainable and resilient food system.

2. <u>Plant-Based Diet and Environmental Impact:</u>

   - Connection with Environment: Embracing a plant-based diet emphasizes the consumption of foods directly derived from the Earth, fostering a deeper connection with nature's abundance.

   - <u>Sustainable Impact:</u>Plant-based diets generally have a lower environmental impact compared to diets rich in animal products, contributing to reduced land use, water consumption, and greenhouse gas emissions.

3. <u>Reducing Food Waste:</u>

   - <u>Connection with Environment:</u> Mindful eating involves appreciating the value of each meal and ingredient, promoting a greater awareness of food resources.

- <u>Sustainable Impact:</u> Minimizing food waste is a sustainable practice that reduces the environmental impact associated with the production, transportation, and disposal of unused food.

4. <u>Choosing Sustainable Packaging:</u>

   - <u>Connection with Environment:</u> Opting for products with eco-friendly and minimal packaging choices aligns with a conscious approach to consumption.

   - <u>Sustainable Impact:</u> By reducing reliance on single-use plastics and supporting brands with sustainable packaging, individuals contribute to reducing environmental pollution.

5. <u>Supporting Local Farmers and Sustainable Agriculture:</u>

   - <u>Connection with Environment:</u> Engaging with local farmers' markets and community-supported agriculture (CSA) initiatives creates a direct link to the source of food production.

   - <u>Sustainable Impact:</u> Supporting local and sustainable agriculture practices promotes biodiversity, soil health, and overall ecosystem resilience.

6. <u>Mindful Food Choices:</u>

- <u>Connection with Environment</u>: Mindful eating involves making intentional and conscious food choices, recognizing the impact of those choices on personal well-being and the environment.

- <u>Sustainable Impact:</u> By understanding the environmental implications of food choices, individuals can make decisions that align with sustainable and regenerative practices.

7. <u>Reducing Carbon Footprint:</u>

- Connection with Environment: Mindful living includes an awareness of personal impact on the planet. Choosing eco-friendly transportation and reducing energy consumption align with this awareness.

- <u>Sustainable Impact:</u> Reducing carbon footprint contributes to mitigating climate change, aligning with the Mind Diet's emphasis on overall well-being, including the health of the planet.

8. <u>Advocating for Sustainable Policies:</u>

- <u>Connection with Environment:</u> Taking an active stance in advocating for sustainable and environmentally friendly policies demonstrates a commitment to a healthier planet.

- <u>Sustainable Impact:</u> Individual actions can contribute to broader systemic changes, fostering a more sustainable and regenerative approach to food production, distribution, and waste management.

9. <u>Participating in Environmental Initiatives:</u>

- <u>Connection with Environment:</u> Involvement in local environmental initiatives or community gardens provides a hands-on connection to sustainable practices.

- <u>Sustainable Impact:</u> Engaging in community-based environmental efforts fosters a sense of shared responsibility and contributes to positive ecological changes.

<u>Tips for navigating restaurants and social situations as a Mind Diet vegan</u>

Navigating restaurants and social situations as a Mind Diet vegan involves thoughtful planning and effective communication to ensure a positive dining experience. Here are some tips for Mind Diet vegans in various social scenarios:

1. <u>Research Restaurants in Advance:</u>

   - <u>Tip:</u> Before heading to a restaurant, check their menu online to identify vegan-friendly options or dishes that can be easily modified.

   - <u>Benefits:</u> This proactive approach helps you make informed choices and avoids potential frustration when dining out.

2. <u>Call Ahead for Special Requests:</u>

   - <u>Tip:</u> If you have specific dietary needs, consider calling the restaurant in advance to discuss your preferences and inquire about available vegan options.

   - <u>Benefits:</u> This allows the kitchen staff to prepare ahead, ensuring a smoother experience and increasing the likelihood of having a satisfying vegan meal.

3. <u>Be Clear About Dietary Preferences:</u>

- <u>Tip:</u> Clearly communicate your dietary preferences to the server, specifying that you follow a vegan Mind Diet and explaining any restrictions or modifications needed.

- <u>Benefits:</u> This helps avoid misunderstandings and ensures that your meal aligns with your nutritional goals.

4. <u>Customize Your Order:</u>

- <u>Tip:</u> Don't hesitate to customize menu items by requesting plant-based substitutions or alterations to meet your Mind Diet preferences.

- <u>Benefits:</u> Most restaurants are willing to accommodate dietary preferences, and customizing your order ensures you get a well-balanced vegan meal.

5. <u>Scan the Entire Menu:</u>

- <u>Tip:</u> Even if there isn't a designated vegan section, look through the entire menu for potential plant-based options or components that can be combined to create a satisfying meal.

- <u>Benefits:</u> This expands your choices and increases the likelihood of finding a diverse and nutritionally rich option.

6. <u>Ask About Ingredients:</u>

- Tip: If uncertain about the ingredients in a dish, don't hesitate to ask the server or kitchen staff for clarification.

- Benefits: This ensures you avoid non-vegan ingredients and aligns with the Mind Diet's focus on conscious and mindful food choices.

7. Be Gracious and Patient:

- Tip: Approach restaurant staff with kindness and patience, recognizing that not all establishments may be familiar with vegan Mind Diet preferences.

- Benefits: A positive and understanding attitude fosters cooperation and may lead to a more enjoyable dining experience.

8. Explore Ethnic Cuisines:

- Tip: Consider exploring ethnic cuisines known for their plant-based options, such as Mediterranean, Indian, or Thai restaurants.

- Benefits: These cuisines often feature diverse and flavorful vegan dishes that align well with the Mind Diet principles.

9. Bring Vegan Snacks:

- Tip: If attending a social gathering with uncertain food options, bring a few vegan snacks or a small dish to share, ensuring you have something to enjoy.

- <u>Benefits:</u> This proactive step ensures you won't go hungry and may introduce others to delicious plant-based options.

10. <u>Educate and Share:</u>

- <u>Tip:</u> Take the opportunity to educate friends or family about the Mind Diet and why you've chosen a vegan approach.

- <u>Benefits:</u> Sharing your perspective can create understanding and may lead to more inclusive and accommodating social gatherings.

11. <u>Check for Vegan-Friendly Restaurants:</u>

- <u>Tip:</u> Explore apps or websites that identify vegan-friendly restaurants in your area. These resources can simplify the process of finding suitable dining options.

- <u>Benefits:</u> Vegan-friendly platforms provide a curated list of establishments, saving you time and effort in your search.

12. <u>Plan Ahead for Events:</u>

- <u>Tip:</u> If attending events with catered meals, reach out to organizers in advance to communicate your dietary preferences and ensure there are suitable vegan options.

- <u>Benefits:</u> This proactive approach helps event organizers accommodate your needs and ensures a more enjoyable experience.

<u>Recommendations for making informed choices when dining out</u>

Making informed choices when dining out as a Mind Diet vegan involves a combination of preparation, communication, and mindfulness to ensure a satisfying and nutritionally balanced meal. Here are recommendations to help Mind Diet vegans make informed choices when dining out:

1. <u>Review Menus in Advance:</u>

   - <u>Recommendation:</u> Take the time to review restaurant menus online before heading out. Look for plant-based options or dishes that can be modified to fit your Mind Diet preferences.

   - <u>Benefits:</u> This proactive step helps you make informed choices and minimizes potential challenges when deciding on a meal at the restaurant.

2. <u>Communicate Dietary Preferences Clearly:</u>

   - <u>Recommendation:</u> Clearly communicate your vegan Mind Diet preferences to the server. Specify any restrictions or modifications needed for your meal.

- <u>Benefits:</u> Effective communication ensures that your dietary needs are understood by the restaurant staff, leading to a more satisfying dining experience.

3. <u>Ask Questions About Ingredients and Preparation:</u>

- <u>Recommendation:</u> Don't hesitate to ask questions about the ingredients used in dishes and how they are prepared. This ensures you avoid non-vegan components and make choices aligned with the Mind Diet.

- <u>Benefits:</u> Understanding the preparation methods helps you make informed decisions about the nutritional content of your meal.

4. <u>Customize Your Order:</u>

- <u>Recommendation:</u> Take advantage of the opportunity to customize your order. Many restaurants are willing to accommodate dietary preferences, such as substituting animal products with plant-based alternatives.

- <u>Benefits:</u> Customizing your order allows you to create a well-balanced and satisfying vegan meal that aligns with the Mind Diet principles.

5. <u>Explore Side Dishes and Appetizers:</u>

- <u>Recommendation</u>: Explore the side dishes and appetizer sections of the menu, as they often feature plant-based options or components that can be combined for a satisfying meal.

- <u>Benefits:</u> This expands your choices and provides an opportunity to create a diverse and nutritionally rich plate.

6. <u>Inquire About Vegan-Friendly Cooking Methods:</u>

- <u>Recommendation:</u> Ask about the cooking methods used in the restaurant. Opt for options that involve grilling, roasting, sautéing in vegetable broth, or other plant-based cooking techniques.

- <u>Benefits:</u> Choosing vegan-friendly cooking methods enhances the flavors of plant-based dishes while aligning with the Mind Diet's focus on mindful and nutritious choices.

7. <u>Be Wary of Hidden Ingredients:</u>

- <u>Recommendation:</u> Be aware of hidden animal-derived ingredients, such as broths, sauces, or dressings. Ask for clarifications to ensure your meal is entirely plant-based.

- <u>Benefits:</u> Avoiding hidden animal products supports your commitment to a vegan Mind Diet and prevents unintended consumption of non-vegan components.

8. Seek Out Vegan-Friendly Restaurants:

   - Recommendation: Explore restaurants known for their vegan-friendly options. Apps or websites that curate such information can simplify the process of finding suitable dining establishments.

   - Benefits: Vegan-friendly restaurants offer a higher likelihood of diverse and well-prepared plant-based choices that align with Mind Diet principles.

9. Order Mindfully at Fast Food Chains:

   - Recommendation: When dining at fast-food chains, research and choose vegan options or customize existing items to suit your Mind Diet preferences.

   - Benefits: Even in fast-food settings, you can make mindful choices by selecting plant-based options and avoiding non-vegan ingredients.

10. Plan for Social Events:

   - Recommendation: If attending social events or gatherings, communicate your dietary preferences to organizers in advance. This ensures there are suitable vegan options available.

   - Benefits: Proactive communication helps create a more inclusive dining experience, aligning with the Mind Diet's focus on well-being in social situations.

11. <u>Express Gratitude for Accommodations:</u>

- <u>Recommendation:</u> Express gratitude to the restaurant staff for accommodating your dietary preferences. Positive interactions foster understanding and may contribute to a more vegan-friendly dining environment.

- <u>Benefits:</u> Acknowledging efforts encourages a positive relationship between Mind Diet vegans and restaurant establishments.

Chapter 12: Mindfulness Practices Beyond Food

Integrating mindfulness into daily routines

Integrating mindfulness into daily routines is a powerful complement to the Mind Diet for vegans, fostering a holistic approach to well-being that encompasses mental, emotional, and physical health. Here are ways Mind Diet vegans can infuse mindfulness into their daily lives:

1. Mindful Meal Preparation:

   - Integration: Engage in mindful meal preparation by focusing on each step of the cooking process. Pay attention to colors, textures, and aromas of ingredients.

   - Benefits: This practice not only enhances the culinary experience but also encourages a deeper connection with the nourishing qualities of plant-based foods.

2. Conscious Eating Habits:

   - Integration: Practice mindful eating by savoring each bite, chewing slowly, and paying attention to flavors and textures. Eliminate distractions during meals.

   - Benefits: Mindful eating promotes better digestion, reduces overeating, and allows Mind Diet vegans to fully appreciate the sensory aspects of their plant-based meals.

3. <u>Morning Meditation or Mindful Breathing:</u>

   - <u>Integration:</u> Start the day with a short meditation or mindful breathing exercise. Focus on the breath to cultivate a sense of calm and presence.

   - <u>Benefits:</u> Morning mindfulness sets a positive tone for the day, promoting mental clarity and emotional resilience.

4. <u>Nature Connection:</u>

   - <u>Integration:</u> Spend time outdoors, whether it's a walk in a park or simply appreciating natural surroundings. Observe the beauty of the environment.

   - <u>Benefits:</u> Connecting with nature enhances overall well-being, aligning with the Mind Diet's holistic approach to health.

5. <u>Gratitude Practice:</u>

   - <u>Integration:</u> Incorporate a daily gratitude practice, reflecting on the positive aspects of life. Consider expressing gratitude for the nourishing plant-based foods you consume.

   - <u>Benefits:</u> Cultivating gratitude fosters a positive mindset and contributes to mental and emotional well-being.

6. <u>Mindful Movement:</u>

- Integration: Choose mindful movement practices such as yoga or tai chi. Focus on the sensations in your body and the connection between movement and breath.

- Benefits: Mindful movement enhances flexibility, strength, and mental clarity, complementing the physical benefits of the Mind Diet.

7. Mindful Snacking:

- Integration: When snacking, be mindful of portion sizes and the flavors of the food. Avoid eating while distracted and savor each bite.

- Benefits: Mindful snacking helps prevent overconsumption and promotes a more conscious relationship with food.

8. Mindful Hydration:

- Integration: Practice mindfulness while hydrating by fully experiencing the act of drinking water. Pay attention to the sensation of hydration and the refreshment it provides.

- Benefits: This simple practice reinforces a mindful approach to self-care and ensures adequate hydration, supporting overall health.

9. Technology Detox:

- <u>Integration</u>: Dedicate specific times for a technology detox. Disconnect from screens, social media, and notifications to create moments of mindfulness.

- <u>Benefits</u>: Technology breaks enhance present-moment awareness and reduce mental clutter, promoting a more focused and centered mindset.

10. <u>Mindful Evening Reflection</u>:

- <u>Integration</u>: Before bedtime, engage in a mindful reflection on the day. Acknowledge achievements, express gratitude, and let go of any stress or tension.

- <u>Benefits</u>: This practice supports restful sleep and prepares the mind for the next day, contributing to overall mental well-being.

11. <u>Mindful Social Interactions</u>:

- <u>Integration</u>: Approach social interactions with mindfulness. Fully engage in conversations, practice active listening, and be present with others.

- <u>Benefits</u>: Mindful social interactions foster meaningful connections and contribute to positive mental and emotional states.

12. <u>Evening Relaxation Rituals</u>:

- Integration: Establish calming evening rituals such as gentle stretching, reading, or practicing relaxation techniques. Create a serene environment to unwind.

- Benefits: Mindful relaxation rituals prepare the mind for restful sleep, supporting mental and emotional balance.

<u>Exploring complementary practices such as meditation and stress reduction</u>

Exploring complementary practices like meditation and stress reduction can greatly enhance the benefits of the Mind Diet for vegans. These practices contribute to overall well-being by addressing mental and emotional aspects, complementing the physical benefits derived from a plant-based diet. Here's how Mind Diet vegans can incorporate meditation and stress reduction into their lifestyle:

1. <u>Mindful Meditation:</u>

- Integration: Establish a daily mindful meditation practice. Focus on the breath, sensations, or guided meditations that align with the Mind Diet's holistic approach to well-being.

- Benefits: Mindful meditation enhances mental clarity, reduces stress, and promotes emotional balance, creating synergy with the cognitive health goals of the Mind Diet.

2. <u>Breathing Exercises:</u>

   - <u>Integration:</u> Incorporate simple breathing exercises into your daily routine. Techniques like deep breathing or diaphragmatic breathing can be done anywhere, promoting relaxation.

   - <u>Benefits:</u> Controlled breathing reduces stress, enhances oxygenation, and supports overall cognitive function, complementing the Mind Diet's focus on brain health.

3. <u>Yoga for Stress Reduction:</u>

   - <u>Integration:</u> Engage in regular yoga sessions. Choose styles emphasizing relaxation, such as Yin or Restorative yoga, to reduce stress and promote flexibility.

   - <u>Benefits:</u> Yoga combines mindful movement with breath awareness, fostering stress reduction and contributing to a calm and centered mindset.

4. <u>Guided Imagery and Visualization:</u>

   - <u>Integration:</u> Practice guided imagery or visualization exercises to create mental images promoting relaxation and positive emotions.

- <u>Benefits:</u> Visualization techniques help reduce stress, anxiety, and support mental resilience, aligning with the Mind Diet's holistic approach to cognitive health.

5. <u>Progressive Muscle Relaxation:</u>

- <u>Integration:</u> Incorporate progressive muscle relaxation techniques into your routine. Gradually tense and release muscle groups to alleviate physical and mental tension.

- <u>Benefits:</u> Progressive muscle relaxation contributes to stress reduction, improves sleep, and complements the Mind Diet's emphasis on overall well-being.

6. <u>Mindful Walking:</u>

- <u>Integration:</u> Practice mindful walking by paying attention to each step, the sensations in your body, and your surroundings. This can be done outdoors or indoors.

- <u>Benefits:</u> Mindful walking serves as a moving meditation, promoting stress reduction and grounding your awareness in the present moment.

7. <u>Body Scan Meditation:</u>

- Integration: Incorporate body scan meditations where you systematically focus on different parts of your body, releasing tension and promoting relaxation.

- Benefits: Body scan meditations enhance body awareness, reduce physical tension, and contribute to a sense of calm and mindfulness.

8. Nature Connection and Mindfulness:

- Integration: Spend time in nature with a mindful approach. Observe the sights, sounds, and sensations around you, fostering a sense of connection and tranquility.

- Benefits: Nature mindfulness practices promote stress reduction, enhance mood, and align with the Mind Diet's holistic perspective on well-being.

9. Journaling for Stress Release:

- Integration: Establish a journaling practice to express thoughts and emotions. Use reflective prompts or gratitude journaling to cultivate a positive mindset.

- Benefits: Journaling serves as a therapeutic outlet, supporting emotional well-being and providing clarity, which complements the Mind Diet's focus on cognitive health.

10. Mindfulness-Based Stress Reduction (MBSR) Programs:

- Integration: Explore mindfulness-based stress reduction programs. These structured courses often include meditation, yoga, and mindful awareness practices.

- Benefits: MBSR programs are designed to reduce stress, enhance well-being, and provide a framework that aligns with the Mind Diet's comprehensive approach to health.

11. Digital Detox and Mindful Technology Use:

- Integration: Implement digital detox periods to reduce screen time and mindfully engage with technology. Set boundaries to prevent constant connectivity-related stress.

- Benefits: Mindful technology use contributes to stress reduction, supports better sleep, and fosters a healthier relationship with digital devices.

12. Mindfulness-Based Cognitive Therapy (MBCT):

- Integration: Explore mindfulness-based cognitive therapy, which combines mindfulness practices with cognitive-behavioral techniques. It is designed to reduce stress and prevent relapses of mental health conditions.

- Benefits: MBCT provides tools for managing stress, promoting emotional resilience, and aligns with the Mind Diet's emphasis on comprehensive well-being.